Copyright © 2023 by Lily J. Thompson (Author)

This book is protected by copyright law and is intended solely for personal use. Reproduction, distribution, or any other form of use requires the written permission of the author. The information presented in this book is for educational and entertainment purposes only, and while every effort has been made to ensure its accuracy and completeness, no guarantees are made. The author is not providing legal, financial, medical, or professional advice, and readers should consult with a licensed professional before implementing any of the techniques discussed in this book. The content in this book has been sourced from various reliable sources, but readers should exercise their own judgment when using this information. The author is not responsible for any losses, direct or indirect, that may occur from the use of this book, including but not limited to errors, omissions, or inaccuracies.

We hope this book has been informative and helpful on your journey to understanding and celebrating older adults. Thank you for your interest and support!

Title: Embracing Aging-A Guide to Understanding and Celebrating Older Adults
Subtitle: Discovering the Beauty and Wisdom of Growing Old with Grace and Dignity

Series: Golden Living: A Guide to Aging Well Clues in the Community

By Lily J. Thompson

Table of Contents

Introduction 6
Defining the concept of "elder" and why it's important to understand aging and older adults 6
The scope of the book and its relevance to readers of all ages and backgrounds 8
Preview of the topics covered in the book 10

Chapter 1: The Aging Process 12
Overview of how the body and mind change as we age . 12
The role of genetics, lifestyle, and environment in the aging process 14
Common health issues and conditions that affect older adults 16
The impact of aging on social and psychological well-being 19

Chapter 2: Bridging the Generational Divide 21
Understanding the differences and similarities between generations 21
Communicating effectively with older adults 24
Developing empathy and respect for seniors 26
Building intergenerational connections and relationships 28

Chapter 3: Aging in America 32

Demographic trends and statistics related to aging in the United States 32
Economic, social, and political factors that affect the lives of older Americans 34
Challenges and opportunities associated with aging in America 38
Policies and programs that support aging in place and promote healthy aging 41

Chapter 4: Aging Around the World 46
International perspectives on aging and older adults 46
Cultural attitudes and beliefs about aging 49
Comparative analysis of policies and programs related to aging in different countries 50
Global trends and challenges related to aging populations 53

Chapter 5: Appreciating the Beauty and Wisdom of Aging 55
Challenging stereotypes and ageism 55
The value of intergenerational learning and knowledge sharing 57
The benefits of aging, including greater wisdom, resilience, and creativity 60
Strategies for celebrating and embracing the aging process 62

Chapter 6: Building Healthy Habits and Relationships in Later Life 65
   The importance of physical and mental health in aging 65
   Strategies for staying active and engaged 70
   Maintaining social connections and relationships 72
   Planning for end-of-life care and decisions 75
Conclusion 77
   Summary of key takeaways from the book 77
   Reflection on the significance of understanding aging and older adults 80
   Call to action for readers to engage with and support the elder population in their communities 83
Key Terms and Definitions 86
Supporting Materials 88

Introduction
Defining the concept of "elder" and why it's important to understand aging and older adults

As we grow older, we become part of a unique demographic known as "elders." Although the definition of an elder may vary depending on culture and context, it generally refers to individuals who have reached a certain age and have experienced the physical, social, and psychological changes associated with aging.

It is important to understand the concept of elderhood and aging because it affects us all in some way. Whether we are approaching old age ourselves or have elderly loved ones, aging is an inevitable part of life that can impact our health, relationships, and overall well-being.

As we age, our bodies and minds undergo significant changes. Physical changes such as wrinkles, gray hair, and decreased mobility are visible signs of aging, but there are also internal changes that are less noticeable. Our cells, tissues, and organs gradually lose function, leading to a decline in physical health. At the same time, our brains undergo structural and functional changes that affect memory, cognition, and emotions.

In addition to physical changes, aging also impacts our social and psychological well-being. Many older adults experience loneliness, social isolation, and ageism, which can negatively impact mental health and quality of life. However, aging also brings opportunities for growth and wisdom, as well as the potential for intergenerational connections and learning.

Understanding the concept of elderhood and aging can also help us appreciate the contributions and experiences of older adults. Older individuals have lived through significant historical events, social changes, and personal experiences that provide unique insights and perspectives. Recognizing the value of these experiences can help promote respect and empathy for older adults.

Overall, the concept of elderhood and aging is complex and multifaceted, encompassing physical, social, and psychological changes. By understanding and appreciating the aging process, we can better support and empower older adults to live healthy and fulfilling lives.

The scope of the book and its relevance to readers of all ages and backgrounds

The scope of this book is broad, as it aims to provide readers of all ages and backgrounds with a comprehensive understanding of aging and older adults. Whether you are a senior citizen, a caregiver, a family member, a healthcare professional, or simply interested in the subject, this book has something to offer.

The book covers a wide range of topics related to aging, including the aging process, social and psychological well-being, bridging the generational divide, policies and programs related to aging in America and around the world, the benefits of aging, and strategies for building healthy habits and relationships in later life. Each chapter is designed to be accessible and informative, with a mix of research-based information, personal stories, and practical tips.

One of the key goals of this book is to challenge ageism and promote positive attitudes towards aging and older adults. Too often, older adults are stereotyped and marginalized, with their experiences and contributions to society overlooked. This book seeks to celebrate the beauty and wisdom of aging, and to demonstrate how older adults can continue to lead fulfilling and meaningful lives.

Another important theme of this book is the importance of intergenerational connections and relationships. Whether it is between family members, neighbors, or members of the larger community, these relationships have the potential to enrich our lives and promote mutual understanding and respect. The book provides practical advice on how to build and maintain these connections, and highlights the benefits of intergenerational learning and knowledge sharing.

Ultimately, this book is intended to be a resource for anyone interested in aging and older adults. By providing a comprehensive overview of the subject, along with practical tips and personal stories, the book aims to promote greater understanding and appreciation of this important stage of life.

Preview of the topics covered in the book

In this book, we will explore the aging process and what it means to grow old with grace and dignity. We will delve into the physical and psychological changes that occur as we age, the social and economic challenges faced by older adults, and the many joys and benefits of aging.

Chapter 1 will provide an overview of the aging process, including how the body and mind change as we age, and the role of genetics, lifestyle, and environment in the aging process. We will also discuss common health issues and conditions that affect older adults and the impact of aging on social and psychological well-being.

Chapter 2 will focus on bridging the generational divide and developing empathy and respect for seniors. We will explore effective communication strategies and ways to build intergenerational connections and relationships.

In Chapter 3, we will take a closer look at aging in America, including demographic trends and statistics related to aging, economic, social, and political factors that affect the lives of older Americans, challenges and opportunities associated with aging in America, and policies and programs that support aging in place and promote healthy aging.

Chapter 4 will broaden our perspective on aging by exploring international perspectives on aging and older adults, cultural attitudes and beliefs about aging, comparative analysis of policies and programs related to aging in different countries, and global trends and challenges related to aging populations.

Chapter 5 will challenge stereotypes and ageism and highlight the value of intergenerational learning and knowledge sharing. We will discuss the benefits of aging, including greater wisdom, resilience, and creativity, and strategies for celebrating and embracing the aging process.

In Chapter 6, we will focus on building healthy habits and relationships in later life. We will discuss the importance of physical and mental health in aging, strategies for staying active and engaged, maintaining social connections and relationships, and planning for end-of-life care and decisions.

In the conclusion, we will summarize the key takeaways from the book, reflect on the significance of understanding aging and older adults, and issue a call to action for readers to engage with and support the elder population in their communities.

Through this comprehensive exploration of aging and older adults, readers of all ages and backgrounds will gain a deeper understanding and appreciation of the beauty and wisdom of growing old with grace and dignity.

Chapter 1: The Aging Process
Overview of how the body and mind change as we age

As we age, our bodies and minds undergo a gradual and complex process of change. These changes can affect our physical health, cognitive abilities, and emotional well-being. In this chapter, we will explore the different ways in which aging can impact our bodies and minds.

Physical Changes: One of the most visible changes that occur as we age is in our physical appearance. Skin loses elasticity, and wrinkles may appear. Hair may become thin and gray, and nails may become brittle. However, the changes that occur beneath the surface of our skin can be much more significant. As we age, our bones can become weaker and more brittle, leading to an increased risk of fractures. Our muscles also tend to lose strength and mass, which can impact our balance, flexibility, and mobility. Additionally, our vision and hearing may become less acute, and our immune system may weaken, making us more vulnerable to infections and illnesses.

Cognitive Changes: Aging can also impact our cognitive abilities. While some changes, such as a decline in processing speed and working memory, are a natural part of the aging process, others may be the result of underlying health conditions or medication use. For example, older adults may experience a decline in their ability to learn and remember new information, or they may have difficulty with tasks that require multitasking or problem-solving. However, research has shown that many older adults are able to compensate for these cognitive changes by relying on their accumulated knowledge and life experience.

Emotional Changes: Aging can also impact our emotional well-being. While many older adults report feeling happier and more content with life than they did in their younger years, others may experience feelings of sadness, loneliness, or anxiety. These emotions may be related to physical health problems, cognitive changes, or social isolation. It's important to address these emotional changes and seek support from friends, family members, or mental health professionals when needed.

In summary, aging is a multifaceted process that affects our bodies and minds in many different ways. By understanding these changes, we can take steps to promote our physical, cognitive, and emotional health as we age.

The role of genetics, lifestyle, and environment in the aging process

The aging process is a complex interplay of various factors, including genetics, lifestyle, and environment. While our genes determine the basic blueprint of our bodies, it's important to note that they're not the only factors that contribute to how we age. Lifestyle choices and environmental factors can also have a significant impact on our health and well-being as we grow older.

Genetics plays a crucial role in determining how we age. Certain genes have been linked to longevity, while others may predispose individuals to specific health conditions or diseases. However, it's important to note that genetic predisposition doesn't necessarily mean that a person will develop a particular condition. Lifestyle choices and environmental factors can either exacerbate or mitigate the effects of our genes.

For instance, smoking, poor diet, lack of exercise, and excessive alcohol consumption are all lifestyle factors that have been linked to a higher risk of developing chronic conditions such as heart disease, diabetes, and cancer. On the other hand, adopting a healthy lifestyle that includes regular physical activity, a balanced diet, and stress management can help slow down the aging process and prevent or manage chronic conditions.

In addition to lifestyle choices, environmental factors such as air pollution, exposure to toxins, and social isolation can also contribute to accelerated aging. For example, studies have shown that living in areas with high levels of air pollution can increase the risk of cognitive decline and Alzheimer's disease. Similarly, social isolation and loneliness have been linked to a higher risk of developing chronic diseases and premature mortality.

Therefore, it's crucial to understand the role that genetics, lifestyle, and environment play in the aging process. By adopting healthy lifestyle choices, minimizing exposure to environmental toxins, and cultivating social connections, individuals can take proactive steps to maintain their health and well-being as they age.

Common health issues and conditions that affect older adults

As we age, our bodies and minds undergo a variety of changes that can lead to health issues and conditions. In this chapter, we will explore some of the most common health issues and conditions that affect older adults.

1. Arthritis: Arthritis is a common condition that affects the joints and causes pain and inflammation. As we age, our risk of developing arthritis increases due to the wear and tear on our joints over time.

2. Osteoporosis: Osteoporosis is a condition in which bones become weak and brittle, making them more prone to fractures. Women are at higher risk of developing osteoporosis, especially after menopause.

3. Cardiovascular disease: Cardiovascular disease is a term that encompasses a range of conditions that affect the heart and blood vessels, including high blood pressure, heart disease, and stroke. Our risk of developing cardiovascular disease increases as we age, but there are many lifestyle changes that can help to prevent it.

4. Diabetes: Diabetes is a condition in which the body is unable to properly regulate blood sugar levels. Type 2 diabetes is more common in older adults and can be managed through diet and exercise.

5. Dementia: Dementia is a group of conditions that affect cognitive function, including memory, thinking, and communication. Alzheimer's disease is the most common form of dementia, and it affects millions of older adults worldwide.

6. Depression: Depression is a common condition that can affect people of all ages, but it is more prevalent in older adults. It can be caused by a variety of factors, including social isolation, chronic illness, and changes in brain chemistry.

7. Falls: Falls are a common cause of injury and hospitalization among older adults. As we age, our balance and coordination can decline, making us more prone to falls. There are many steps that can be taken to reduce the risk of falls, including regular exercise and making changes to the home environment.

8. Hearing and vision loss: Hearing and vision loss are common as we age, and they can have a significant impact on our quality of life. Regular screenings and early treatment can help to prevent or manage these conditions.

In this chapter, we have provided an overview of some of the most common health issues and conditions that affect older adults. It's important to note that everyone's experience with aging is unique, and there are many factors that can impact our health and well-being. However, by understanding these common health issues and conditions, we can take steps to prevent or manage them and maintain our health and independence as we age.

The impact of aging on social and psychological well-being

As we age, not only do our bodies change, but our social and psychological well-being is also significantly affected. This chapter will explore the various ways aging can impact our social and psychological health.

Firstly, let's consider the social aspect of aging. As we age, we may face changes in our social lives, such as retirement, loss of loved ones, and declining physical health. These changes can lead to social isolation and loneliness, which in turn can have negative impacts on our mental and physical health. Social isolation has been linked to depression, anxiety, and cognitive decline in older adults.

It's important to note that social support can have a significant positive impact on older adults' well-being. Having close relationships with family and friends, engaging in social activities, and participating in community groups can promote social connectedness and improve overall quality of life. In fact, studies have shown that social support can lead to a reduced risk of depression, cognitive decline, and even mortality in older adults.

Moving on to the psychological impacts of aging, older adults may experience changes in cognitive abilities, such as memory and attention span. While these changes are a natural part of the aging process, they can still be challenging for some individuals. Additionally, older adults may face mental health challenges such as depression and anxiety, which can be exacerbated by social isolation and physical health problems.

However, it's not all negative. As we age, we may also develop greater emotional maturity, resilience, and self-awareness. Older adults may also have a more positive outlook on life, and a greater sense of purpose and meaning. Studies have shown that older adults who maintain a positive attitude towards aging have better physical and mental health outcomes than those who view aging negatively.

In conclusion, the impact of aging on social and psychological well-being is complex and multifaceted. While there may be challenges associated with aging, it's important to recognize the positive aspects and take steps to promote social connectedness, mental health, and emotional well-being in older adults.

Chapter 2: Bridging the Generational Divide
Understanding the differences and similarities between generations

Understanding the differences and similarities between generations is essential for building meaningful relationships and effective communication with older adults. Generational differences can shape attitudes, beliefs, values, and behaviors, and understanding these differences can help us appreciate and respect diverse perspectives.

One of the most significant differences between generations is their attitudes towards technology. While younger generations have grown up with technology and are often referred to as "digital natives," older adults may struggle with using new technologies, such as smartphones, social media, and other digital platforms. However, this does not mean that older adults are not interested in technology. In fact, many seniors are eager to learn and embrace new technologies, and it's important to provide them with opportunities and support to do so.

Another difference between generations is their approach to work and career. Baby Boomers, for example, may have a more traditional approach to work, valuing stability, loyalty, and career advancement. In contrast, younger generations may prioritize work-life balance, flexibility, and fulfillment over traditional notions of career success. Understanding these differences can help managers and employers create more inclusive and supportive work environments that meet the needs and expectations of workers from different generations.

Another important factor to consider is the historical and social context in which each generation grew up. Baby Boomers, for example, grew up during a time of significant social and political change, such as the Civil Rights Movement and the Vietnam War. This context shaped their attitudes and values towards issues such as race, gender, and social justice. Similarly, younger generations have grown up in a time of technological and social change, which has influenced their attitudes and beliefs towards issues such as diversity, inclusion, and sustainability.

To bridge the generational divide, it's important to approach interactions with older adults with empathy, respect, and openness. This means being patient and understanding of their unique experiences and perspectives, while also being willing to learn and adapt to their needs and preferences. It also means being aware of our own assumptions and biases towards older adults, and challenging stereotypes and ageism in ourselves and others.

In summary, understanding the differences and similarities between generations is essential for building meaningful relationships and effective communication with older adults. By recognizing and appreciating diverse perspectives, we can bridge generational divides and create more inclusive and supportive communities for people of all ages.

Communicating effectively with older adults

Communicating effectively with older adults is an important skill that can enhance relationships and facilitate understanding between generations. However, it can be challenging due to potential differences in language, culture, and experiences. In this section, we will explore strategies for effective communication with older adults.

1. Be Patient and Listen Attentively Communication with older adults can take longer and require more patience. It is important to listen attentively to what they have to say and allow them enough time to express their thoughts.

2. Use Clear and Simple Language Using clear and simple language is essential when communicating with older adults, especially those with hearing or cognitive impairments. Avoid using jargon or technical terms that they may not understand.

3. Avoid Stereotypes and Assumptions Stereotypes and assumptions can create barriers in communication. It is important to avoid making assumptions based on age or other characteristics and treat older adults as individuals with unique experiences and perspectives.

4. Show Respect and Empathy Older adults have a wealth of knowledge and experience that should be

respected. Show empathy and respect for their feelings and experiences, even if they differ from your own.

5. Use Non-Verbal Communication Non-verbal communication, such as facial expressions and body language, can be just as important as verbal communication. Pay attention to non-verbal cues and use them to help you better understand the older adult's perspective.

6. Provide Visual Aids Visual aids, such as pictures or diagrams, can be helpful in communicating complex ideas or concepts. They can also be useful for individuals with hearing or cognitive impairments.

7. Allow for Two-Way Communication Effective communication is a two-way process. Allow older adults to ask questions and express their own thoughts and feelings. This can help to build trust and understanding between generations.

By employing these strategies, you can communicate more effectively with older adults, enhance your relationships, and gain a better understanding of their perspectives and experiences.

Developing empathy and respect for seniors

Developing empathy and respect for seniors is essential in bridging the generational divide. Seniors are often overlooked, undervalued, and marginalized in society, leading to a lack of understanding and respect for their experiences and perspectives. This can create barriers to effective communication and hinder meaningful relationships between generations. Developing empathy and respect for seniors involves understanding and valuing their unique life experiences, perspectives, and contributions to society.

One of the key ways to develop empathy and respect for seniors is to actively listen to their stories and experiences. Seniors have a wealth of knowledge and life experience that can be shared and learned from. By taking the time to listen to their stories, we can gain a better understanding of their perspectives, values, and beliefs. This can help us develop a deeper respect and appreciation for their contributions and experiences.

Another way to develop empathy and respect for seniors is to challenge ageist attitudes and stereotypes. Ageism is a pervasive form of discrimination that can lead to negative perceptions and assumptions about older adults. By challenging ageist attitudes and stereotypes, we can promote a more positive and respectful image of seniors in society. This can help break down barriers between generations and foster more meaningful relationships.

It is also important to recognize and acknowledge the unique challenges that seniors face. Age-related health issues, financial insecurity, and social isolation are just a few of the challenges that many seniors may experience. By acknowledging these challenges and working to address them, we can show our respect and empathy for the difficulties that seniors may face.

In addition to these actions, it is essential to treat seniors with dignity and respect in our daily interactions. This means showing patience, kindness, and compassion, even in situations that may be frustrating or challenging. By treating seniors with dignity and respect, we can foster a culture of empathy and understanding that can help bridge the generational divide.

In conclusion, developing empathy and respect for seniors is essential in bridging the generational divide. By actively listening to their stories and experiences, challenging ageist attitudes and stereotypes, acknowledging the unique challenges they face, and treating them with dignity and respect, we can promote a more positive and meaningful relationship between generations.

Building intergenerational connections and relationships

One of the most important aspects of bridging the generational divide is the development of intergenerational connections and relationships. By breaking down barriers and fostering understanding and empathy between different age groups, these relationships can provide a range of benefits for all involved.

Benefits of intergenerational connections and relationships

Research has shown that intergenerational connections and relationships can have numerous positive effects on both younger and older individuals. Some of these benefits include:

1. Reduced social isolation: Many older adults experience social isolation and loneliness, which can have negative impacts on both their mental and physical health. Intergenerational relationships can provide opportunities for increased social interaction and a sense of connection with others.

2. Enhanced emotional well-being: Intergenerational relationships can provide a sense of purpose and meaning for older adults, as well as opportunities to share their wisdom and experiences with younger individuals. For

younger individuals, these relationships can provide a sense of guidance and support, as well as exposure to different perspectives and ways of thinking.

3. Improved cognitive function: Interacting with individuals from different age groups can provide opportunities for cognitive stimulation and growth. Older adults who engage in intergenerational relationships have been shown to have better cognitive function and a lower risk of cognitive decline.

4. Increased understanding and empathy: By interacting with individuals from different age groups, people can gain a greater understanding of different life experiences and perspectives. This can lead to increased empathy and a greater appreciation for the contributions of older adults to society.

Strategies for building intergenerational relationships

There are many strategies that can be employed to build intergenerational connections and relationships. Some of these include:

1. Volunteering: Volunteering for organizations or causes that serve people of different ages can provide opportunities for interaction and connection.

2. Participating in community activities: Community events and activities, such as festivals or cultural events, can

provide opportunities for people of different age groups to interact.

3. Mentoring: Older adults can serve as mentors to younger individuals, providing guidance and support in various areas of life.

4. Participating in educational programs: Educational programs, such as lifelong learning classes, can provide opportunities for older adults to interact with younger individuals who share similar interests.

5. Intergenerational living: Housing arrangements that combine different age groups, such as senior living communities that also include young families, can provide opportunities for intergenerational interaction and connection.

In conclusion, building intergenerational connections and relationships is an important step in bridging the generational divide. These relationships can provide numerous benefits for both younger and older individuals, including reduced social isolation, enhanced emotional well-being, improved cognitive function, and increased understanding and empathy. By employing strategies such as volunteering, participating in community activities, mentoring, participating in educational programs, and intergenerational living, individuals can foster these important connections and promote understanding and empathy between different age groups.

Chapter 3: Aging in America
Demographic trends and statistics related to aging in the United States

As the baby boomer generation ages, the United States is experiencing significant demographic shifts. In 2020, there were approximately 54 million Americans aged 65 and older, comprising 16.5% of the total population. By 2030, this number is projected to increase to 73 million, or 21.5% of the total population. By 2050, the number of older Americans is projected to reach 88 million, comprising 22% of the total population.

One of the main drivers of this demographic shift is increased life expectancy. In 1950, the average life expectancy in the United States was 68 years. By 2020, it had increased to 78 years. Furthermore, the number of Americans aged 85 and older is projected to more than triple by 2050, reaching 19 million.

In addition to these demographic trends, there are also significant disparities in aging experiences among different populations. For example, older adults who identify as Black or Hispanic are more likely to live in poverty, experience food insecurity, and have limited access to healthcare. Additionally, LGBTQ older adults often face unique challenges related to discrimination and social isolation.

There are also gender differences in aging experiences. Women live longer than men on average, but they are also more likely to experience poverty and social isolation in later life. Women are also more likely to provide care to family members and therefore may experience greater caregiver stress.

As the population ages, there are also important implications for the labor force and the economy. Older workers are a growing segment of the workforce, with many choosing to work past the traditional retirement age. This trend is partially driven by financial necessity, but also by a desire for social engagement and continued intellectual stimulation. However, age discrimination in the workplace remains a significant challenge for many older workers.

In summary, demographic trends related to aging in the United States are significant and will continue to have far-reaching implications for society as a whole. It is important to understand these trends and their implications in order to better address the needs and challenges facing older Americans.

Economic, social, and political factors that affect the lives of older Americans

Economic, social, and political factors can significantly impact the lives of older Americans. These factors can determine their access to resources, quality of life, and health outcomes. In this section, we will discuss some of the key economic, social, and political factors that affect older Americans.

Economic Factors:

Income and Wealth Inequality: Income and wealth inequality is a significant issue affecting older Americans. According to a report by the Economic Policy Institute, income inequality among older Americans has increased dramatically since the 1980s. This income inequality is due to factors such as changes in pension and retirement plans, the decline of unionization, and the rise of temporary and part-time work. Wealth inequality is another issue affecting older Americans, with the top 10% of older Americans holding over 80% of the wealth.

Social Security: Social Security is a critical program that provides income support to older Americans. It is the primary source of income for many older Americans and provides a safety net for those who have not saved enough for retirement. However, the program is facing financial challenges due to demographic changes, including an aging population and declining birth rates.

Retirement Savings: Retirement savings are an essential factor affecting older Americans' economic well-being. Unfortunately, many older Americans have not saved enough for retirement. A report by the National Institute on Retirement Security found that the median retirement account balance for Americans nearing retirement is just $12,000. This lack of retirement savings is due to a variety of factors, including the decline of traditional pension plans and the rise of individual retirement accounts (IRAs) and 401(k) plans, which require individuals to make their own investment decisions.

Social Factors:

Social Isolation: Social isolation is a significant issue affecting older Americans. According to the AARP, over 8 million older Americans are affected by social isolation. Social isolation can lead to negative health outcomes, including depression, anxiety, and cognitive decline. Social isolation can be caused by a variety of factors, including the loss of friends and family, mobility issues, and the lack of access to transportation.

Ageism: Ageism is another social factor that affects older Americans. Ageism refers to negative attitudes and stereotypes about older adults. Ageism can lead to discrimination in employment, housing, and healthcare. It can also contribute to social isolation and negative health outcomes.

Political Factors:

Healthcare: Healthcare is a critical political issue that affects older Americans. Older Americans have higher healthcare needs than younger Americans and are more likely to have chronic conditions such as diabetes, heart disease, and cancer. Medicare is the primary source of healthcare coverage for older Americans, but the program is facing financial challenges due to rising healthcare costs and an aging population.

Elder Justice: Elder justice is another political issue that affects older Americans. Elder abuse, neglect, and exploitation are significant problems affecting older Americans. According to the National Council on Aging, approximately 1 in 10 Americans over the age of 60 have experienced some form of elder abuse. Elder abuse can lead to negative health outcomes, including depression, anxiety, and cognitive decline. Elder justice advocates are pushing for increased funding for programs and services that protect older Americans from abuse, neglect, and exploitation.

Conclusion:

Economic, social, and political factors significantly impact the lives of older Americans. Income and wealth inequality, social isolation, and ageism are social factors that affect older Americans. Healthcare and elder justice are political issues that affect older Americans. As the population ages, it is critical to address these issues to ensure that older Americans can age with dignity and respect.

Challenges and opportunities associated with aging in America

As the American population continues to age, there are both challenges and opportunities that arise. This chapter will explore the specific challenges that older adults face in America, as well as the opportunities that are available to them.

Challenges

1. Ageism

One of the most significant challenges that older adults face in America is ageism, which is the stereotyping, discrimination, and prejudice against people based on their age. Ageism can lead to negative health outcomes, social isolation, and economic insecurity.

2. Healthcare

Access to affordable and quality healthcare can be a challenge for older Americans, especially those with chronic conditions. The high cost of healthcare, including prescription drugs and long-term care, can be prohibitive for those on fixed incomes.

3. Financial insecurity

Many older Americans face financial insecurity, especially those who rely solely on Social Security benefits for their income. The rising cost of living, including healthcare, housing, and food, can make it difficult for older adults to make ends meet.

4. Social isolation

Social isolation can be a significant problem for older adults, especially those who live alone or have limited mobility. Social isolation can lead to depression, anxiety, and other negative health outcomes.

Opportunities

1. Lifelong learning

One opportunity that older adults have in America is the ability to engage in lifelong learning. Many universities and community colleges offer discounted or free courses for older adults, which can help keep their minds active and engaged.

2. Volunteerism

Volunteerism can be a rewarding opportunity for older adults, as it provides them with a sense of purpose and the ability to give back to their communities. Many organizations, including hospitals, schools, and non-profits, rely on volunteers to carry out their missions.

3. Second careers

With advances in healthcare and technology, many older adults are able to continue working well into their golden years. Starting a second career can be a fulfilling opportunity for older adults who want to continue to be productive and contribute to society.

4. Intergenerational relationships

Building relationships with people of different ages can be a rewarding opportunity for older adults. Interacting with younger generations can help older adults feel connected and valued, while also providing younger people with the opportunity to learn from their wisdom and experience.

Conclusion

While there are certainly challenges associated with aging in America, there are also many opportunities for older adults to live fulfilling and meaningful lives. By addressing the challenges head-on and taking advantage of the opportunities available, older adults can continue to thrive and contribute to society.

Policies and programs that support aging in place and promote healthy aging

As the population of older adults in the United States continues to grow, it is important to understand the policies and programs that support aging in place and promote healthy aging. Aging in place refers to the ability of older adults to remain in their homes and communities as they age, rather than having to move to institutional settings like nursing homes. Promoting healthy aging means enabling older adults to maintain their physical, mental, and social well-being, which can improve their quality of life and reduce healthcare costs.

This chapter will discuss some of the policies and programs that have been developed in the United States to support aging in place and promote healthy aging, as well as some of the challenges associated with implementing these initiatives.

1. The Older Americans Act

The Older Americans Act (OAA) was originally passed by Congress in 1965 and has been reauthorized and amended several times since then. The purpose of the OAA is to support the well-being and independence of older adults by funding a variety of programs and services, such as meal delivery, caregiver support, and transportation. These programs are typically administered at the local level by Area Agencies on Aging (AAAs).

The OAA has been successful in providing critical services to older adults, but there are concerns about the adequacy of funding and the need for more comprehensive services that address the diverse needs of older adults.

2. Medicaid Home and Community-Based Services (HCBS)

Medicaid is a joint federal and state program that provides health insurance for low-income individuals, including many older adults. In addition to covering medical services, Medicaid can also cover Home and Community-Based Services (HCBS), which enable older adults to receive long-term care services in their homes and communities, rather than in institutions like nursing homes.

HCBS can include a range of services, such as personal care assistance, home health care, and adult day care. These services can help older adults maintain their independence and quality of life, but there are concerns about the availability and quality of HCBS, as well as the financial burden that these services can place on older adults and their families.

3. Age-Friendly Communities

Age-Friendly Communities is a movement that started with the World Health Organization (WHO) in 2007 and has since spread to communities throughout the United States. An Age-Friendly Community is one that is designed and adapted to support the physical, social, and emotional well-being of older adults.

Age-Friendly Communities typically focus on making physical environments more accessible and safe, promoting social engagement and inclusion, and improving access to health and community services. These initiatives can improve the health and well-being of older adults, as well as the overall livability of communities.

4. Technology and Aging

Technology is playing an increasingly important role in promoting aging in place and healthy aging. There are a wide variety of technological tools and devices that can enable older adults to remain independent and connected to their communities, such as home monitoring systems, telehealth services, and social media platforms.

However, there are also concerns about the accessibility and affordability of these technologies, as well as the potential for technology to exacerbate social isolation and other challenges associated with aging.

5. Challenges and Opportunities

Despite the various policies and programs that have been developed to support aging in place and healthy aging, there are still many challenges that need to be addressed. These include:
- Financial barriers to accessing services and care
- Lack of access to affordable and accessible housing
- Social isolation and loneliness
- Ageism and discrimination
- Limited availability of culturally appropriate services

Addressing these challenges will require a comprehensive and collaborative approach that involves policymakers, healthcare providers, community organizations, and older adults themselves. However, there are also many opportunities for innovation and progress in this area, such as the increasing availability of technology and telemedicine to support remote healthcare, and the growing recognition of the value of intergenerational programs and initiatives. Additionally, there are a range of policies and programs at the federal, state, and local levels that aim to support aging in place and promote healthy aging, including Medicare and Medicaid, the Older Americans Act, and the Aging and Disability Resource Centers. By understanding these policies and programs, as well as the challenges and opportunities associated with aging in America, we can work towards a future where older adults are able to age with dignity, independence, and access to the resources and support they need.

Chapter 4: Aging Around the World
International perspectives on aging and older adults

Aging is a universal experience that transcends cultural, social, and economic boundaries. While there are similarities in the aging process across different cultures, there are also significant differences in how aging is perceived and experienced around the world. This chapter will explore international perspectives on aging and highlight the unique challenges and opportunities faced by older adults in different parts of the world.

Demographic Trends

The global population is aging at an unprecedented rate, and by 2050, the number of people aged 60 and over is expected to reach 2.1 billion, more than double the number in 2017. This demographic shift is particularly pronounced in developed countries, where falling birth rates and improved healthcare have resulted in an increasingly aging population. However, many developing countries are also experiencing significant increases in life expectancy, which is driving population aging in these regions.

Perceptions of Aging

Cultural attitudes towards aging vary widely across different societies, with some cultures valuing and respecting their elders, while others view old age as a time of decline and irrelevance. In many traditional societies, older adults are regarded as repositories of wisdom and knowledge and play important roles in decision-making and community leadership. However, in other cultures, particularly those with a strong emphasis on youth and physical beauty, older adults may be marginalized and ignored.

Challenges and Opportunities

Older adults face a range of challenges around the world, including poverty, social isolation, and ageism. In many developing countries, older adults may lack access to basic healthcare and social services, and they may be particularly vulnerable to economic instability and political upheaval. However, there are also many opportunities for older adults to lead fulfilling and productive lives, particularly when they are supported by strong social networks and engaged in meaningful activities.

Innovative Approaches

Around the world, there are many innovative approaches to supporting aging populations, ranging from community-based care models to technology-enabled solutions. In some countries, intergenerational living arrangements have been successful in promoting social connectedness and reducing social isolation among older adults. In other regions, mobile health technologies and telemedicine have enabled older adults to access healthcare services remotely, reducing the need for in-person visits and improving health outcomes.

Conclusion

International perspectives on aging highlight the need for culturally sensitive and context-specific approaches to promoting healthy aging and addressing the challenges faced by older adults. By understanding the unique experiences and needs of older adults in different parts of the world, policymakers and healthcare providers can develop more effective strategies for supporting aging populations and promoting healthy aging across the globe.

Cultural attitudes and beliefs about aging

Cultural attitudes and beliefs about aging vary greatly across different parts of the world. In some cultures, older adults are revered and seen as wise and valuable members of society, while in others, they may be marginalized or even disrespected.

For example, in many Asian cultures, respect for elders is deeply ingrained in the society and is considered a core value. Older adults are often seen as keepers of tradition and culture, and their wisdom and life experience are highly valued. In contrast, in Western cultures, youth and vitality are often prized, and aging is sometimes viewed as a negative process to be avoided or minimized.

In some cultures, the family plays a significant role in caring for older adults, with multiple generations often living together in the same household or community. In other cultures, such as in the United States and Western Europe, individualism is highly valued, and older adults may be more likely to live independently or in assisted living facilities.

Cultural attitudes and beliefs about aging can have a significant impact on the way that older adults are treated and cared for in society. Understanding and respecting cultural differences is essential for providing effective and appropriate care for older adults in diverse communities.

Comparative analysis of policies and programs related to aging in different countries

As the world's population ages, many countries are facing similar challenges and opportunities associated with aging. However, each country has its unique cultural, economic, social, and political factors that influence its approach to aging and the elderly. In this chapter, we will compare and contrast policies and programs related to aging in different countries, highlighting their strengths and weaknesses.

One of the countries that have taken a comprehensive approach to aging is Japan. With the highest percentage of elderly people in the world, Japan has developed a wide range of programs and policies that support healthy aging and aging in place. These include long-term care insurance, which provides financial support for in-home care, and universal access to healthcare. Japan also has a strong tradition of intergenerational living, with many families living together in multigenerational households. Additionally, the government has implemented age-friendly initiatives to create more accessible and inclusive environments for older adults.

Another country that has made significant progress in addressing aging-related challenges is Sweden. The Swedish government has long prioritized social welfare policies, including those related to aging. Sweden has a universal healthcare system, and its elderly care services are publicly funded and free of charge. The country also provides extensive support for aging in place, including home modification programs, in-home care services, and transportation assistance. Sweden's social welfare policies have contributed to a high standard of living for its elderly citizens, with one of the highest life expectancies in the world.

In contrast, the United States has a more fragmented approach to aging-related policies and programs. While there are federal programs such as Medicare and Social Security that provide some support for older adults, there is no comprehensive national strategy for addressing aging-related challenges. Instead, policies and programs related to aging are largely the responsibility of individual states and localities. This has resulted in significant disparities in access to healthcare, housing, and social services for older adults across the country.

Other countries, such as China and India, are facing unique challenges related to aging due to their large populations and rapidly changing demographics. In China, the one-child policy has resulted in a shrinking workforce and a rapidly aging population, creating significant economic and social challenges. The Chinese government has responded with policies to support aging in place, including community-based healthcare and in-home care services, as well as age-friendly city initiatives. India, on the other hand, is experiencing a "youth bulge" with a large and growing young population. However, as the country's middle class expands, there is a growing demand for elderly care services and age-friendly environments.

Overall, there is no one-size-fits-all approach to addressing aging-related challenges. Each country's policies and programs must be tailored to its unique cultural, economic, and social context. However, by learning from each other's experiences, countries can develop more effective strategies for promoting healthy aging and aging in place.

Global trends and challenges related to aging populations

As the world's population ages, there are several global trends and challenges related to aging populations that are becoming increasingly prevalent. One of the most significant trends is the increase in the proportion of older adults relative to the overall population, with some countries experiencing more rapid aging than others. This shift in demographics presents several challenges, including increased demand for healthcare and social services, as well as a strain on pension and retirement systems.

Another trend is the growing prevalence of chronic conditions and disabilities, which tend to increase in prevalence with age. This trend is placing additional pressure on healthcare systems and contributing to rising healthcare costs. Additionally, older adults are more likely to experience social isolation and loneliness, which can have negative impacts on their physical and mental health.

The global challenge of aging populations is also compounded by disparities in health outcomes and access to care between different countries and populations. For example, in low- and middle-income countries, older adults are more likely to experience poverty and lack access to healthcare and social services. In contrast, older adults in high-income countries may face the challenges of over-medicalization and over-treatment, as well as social isolation and ageism.

To address these global challenges related to aging populations, policymakers and healthcare systems must prioritize preventative care and social support for older adults. This includes investing in community-based programs that promote healthy aging and address social isolation, as well as ensuring equitable access to healthcare and social services. Collaborative efforts between governments, non-governmental organizations, and the private sector are also necessary to support innovative approaches to addressing the challenges of aging populations around the world.

Chapter 5: Appreciating the Beauty and Wisdom of Aging

Challenging stereotypes and ageism

As we age, we often encounter negative stereotypes and ageism that can impact our mental and physical health. Ageism refers to prejudice or discrimination against individuals based on their age. This prejudice can manifest in many ways, such as assuming older adults are unable to learn new things, discounting their contributions to society, and making assumptions about their health and abilities. These negative stereotypes can have a profound impact on older adults, leading to feelings of isolation, depression, and low self-esteem.

It is important to challenge these stereotypes and negative attitudes towards aging. One way to do this is by promoting positive representations of older adults in media and popular culture. This can include showcasing older adults in a wide range of roles and activities, such as working, volunteering, and pursuing hobbies and interests.

Another way to challenge ageism is by celebrating the wisdom and experience that comes with aging. Older adults have a wealth of knowledge and life experience that can be shared with younger generations. By valuing this wisdom and experience, we can help break down negative stereotypes and promote intergenerational understanding and respect.

Furthermore, it is essential to recognize that aging is a natural part of the human experience and that older adults have value and worth. Ageism can have significant impacts on the mental and physical health of older adults, and it is essential to challenge negative attitudes towards aging to promote healthy aging and positive mental health outcomes.

In conclusion, challenging stereotypes and ageism is crucial to promoting healthy aging and improving the quality of life for older adults. By valuing the wisdom and experience of older adults, promoting positive representations of aging, and recognizing the value and worth of older adults, we can help break down negative stereotypes and promote intergenerational understanding and respect.

The value of intergenerational learning and knowledge sharing

Intergenerational learning and knowledge sharing is an important aspect of appreciating the beauty and wisdom of aging. It involves bringing people from different age groups together to share experiences, skills, and knowledge with each other. This type of learning is beneficial for all involved, as it can help to break down stereotypes, increase understanding, and promote a more positive view of aging.

One of the most significant benefits of intergenerational learning is the opportunity for older adults to share their experiences and wisdom with younger generations. Older adults have a wealth of knowledge and life experience that they can pass down to younger people. This can be particularly valuable in areas such as career development, financial planning, and personal relationships. By sharing their experiences, older adults can help younger people to avoid making the same mistakes and to make more informed decisions.

At the same time, younger people can bring new perspectives and skills to the table, which can be beneficial for older adults. For example, younger people may be more familiar with new technologies and can help older adults to learn how to use them. They may also have fresh ideas and perspectives that can help to challenge stereotypes and promote more positive views of aging.

Intergenerational learning can take many different forms, from formal programs that bring people of different ages together for structured learning experiences, to more informal opportunities for sharing and mentoring. Some examples of intergenerational learning programs include:

1. Mentoring programs: These programs match older adults with younger people who are interested in learning from them. Mentors can provide guidance and support in areas such as career development, financial planning, and personal relationships.

2. Learning circles: These are small groups of people from different age groups who come together to learn from each other. Each person takes a turn sharing something they know or have experienced, and the group discusses and learns from each other.

3. Community service projects: These projects bring people of all ages together to work towards a common goal. For example, a group might work on a community garden or a neighborhood cleanup project.

4. Intergenerational classrooms: These are classrooms that include students of different ages. For example, a school

might pair up younger students with older students to work on a project together.

Overall, intergenerational learning and knowledge sharing is a valuable way to promote understanding and appreciation between different age groups. By bringing people together to share their experiences, skills, and knowledge, we can break down stereotypes and promote a more positive view of aging.

The benefits of aging, including greater wisdom, resilience, and creativity

As people age, they may experience physical and cognitive declines, which can lead to negative stereotypes and beliefs about the aging process. However, there are also many benefits to aging that are often overlooked or undervalued. In this section, we will explore the benefits of aging, including greater wisdom, resilience, and creativity.

Wisdom is often associated with older adults, and for good reason. As people age, they accumulate a wealth of knowledge and life experience that can be invaluable in decision-making and problem-solving. This type of knowledge, often referred to as "crystallized intelligence," involves the ability to use acquired knowledge, skills, and expertise to solve problems and make decisions. Older adults are often better at this type of problem-solving than younger adults because they have had more time to accumulate knowledge and experience.

Resilience is another benefit of aging. Older adults have often faced a variety of challenges throughout their lives, such as loss of loved ones, financial difficulties, and health problems. As a result, they may develop a greater ability to bounce back from setbacks and overcome adversity.

This resilience can be an asset in many areas of life, including personal relationships, work, and health.

Finally, aging can also lead to increased creativity. As people age, they may develop a more nuanced understanding of the world and a deeper appreciation for the beauty of life. This can inspire them to engage in creative pursuits, such as writing, painting, or music. Some studies have even suggested that creativity may continue to improve well into old age.

In addition to these benefits, there are many other ways in which aging can be a positive experience. For example, older adults may have more free time to pursue hobbies and interests, and may also have stronger personal relationships and a greater sense of purpose. By recognizing and valuing the benefits of aging, we can challenge negative stereotypes and create a more positive and inclusive view of the aging process.

Strategies for celebrating and embracing the aging process

As people age, it is important to embrace and celebrate the aging process to live a fulfilling life. Here are some strategies for celebrating and embracing the aging process:

1. Cultivate a positive attitude towards aging: Attitudes towards aging play a significant role in how people experience it. Cultivating a positive attitude towards aging can help people appreciate the benefits of aging and embrace the process. It is important to acknowledge the challenges that come with aging but also focus on the positive aspects.

2. Stay engaged and involved: Being engaged in activities that are personally meaningful and enjoyable can help individuals stay active, happy and healthy. This may include volunteering, joining clubs, attending classes or pursuing hobbies.

3. Practice self-care: Taking care of oneself is important at any age, but it becomes even more crucial as people age. Good self-care habits can help individuals maintain physical and emotional health, including exercise, a healthy diet, adequate sleep, stress reduction techniques, and regular check-ups with healthcare professionals.

4. Maintain social connections: Social isolation and loneliness can be significant problems for older adults, leading to adverse health outcomes. Maintaining social connections with family, friends, and community groups can help individuals stay connected and engaged.

5. Embrace new technologies: Technology can provide opportunities for social connections, learning, and entertainment. Learning new technologies can be a fun and engaging way for older adults to stay connected and engaged.

6. Practice lifelong learning: Lifelong learning is important for personal growth, intellectual stimulation, and overall well-being. Learning can take many forms, including reading, taking courses, attending lectures, and engaging in discussions with peers.

7. Celebrate milestones: Celebrating milestones, such as birthdays or retirements, can be a way to acknowledge and appreciate the achievements and experiences that come with age.

In conclusion, embracing and celebrating the aging process is an important aspect of a fulfilling life. By cultivating a positive attitude towards aging, staying engaged and involved, practicing self-care, maintaining social connections, embracing new technologies, practicing lifelong learning and celebrating milestones, individuals can age gracefully and enjoyably.

Chapter 6: Building Healthy Habits and Relationships in Later Life

The importance of physical and mental health in aging

As people age, it becomes increasingly important to prioritize physical and mental health. Physical health can impact an older adult's ability to live independently, engage in activities they enjoy, and maintain their quality of life. Mental health is also a crucial aspect of overall well-being and can affect an older adult's cognitive function, social connections, and emotional resilience. In this section, we will explore the importance of physical and mental health in aging and discuss strategies for maintaining optimal health.

The Importance of Physical Health in Aging

Physical health is a vital aspect of healthy aging, and maintaining an active lifestyle can help older adults stay healthy and independent. Regular physical activity has been linked to a reduced risk of chronic conditions such as heart disease, stroke, diabetes, and some forms of cancer. Exercise can also help maintain mobility, flexibility, and balance, reducing the risk of falls and injuries.

As people age, their bodies undergo various changes that can impact their physical health. These changes include a decrease in muscle mass, bone density, and flexibility, which can make it more challenging to maintain an active lifestyle. Additionally, chronic health conditions, such as arthritis or chronic pain, can limit physical activity.

Despite these challenges, older adults can still engage in physical activity to maintain their health. Exercise programs that focus on improving strength, balance, and flexibility can help older adults maintain their physical function and reduce their risk of falls. Physical activity can also have mental health benefits, such as reducing stress and improving mood.

The Importance of Mental Health in Aging

Mental health is an essential component of overall well-being, and older adults may be at risk for mental health conditions such as depression and anxiety. According to the National Institute of Mental Health, depression affects more than 2 million older adults in the United States. Older adults may also experience anxiety related to social isolation, loss of independence, or chronic health conditions.

Maintaining mental health in aging involves a variety of strategies, including staying socially engaged, maintaining cognitive function, and seeking professional support when needed. Social engagement can help prevent loneliness and isolation, which can have negative impacts on mental health. Maintaining cognitive function, such as through engaging in mental exercises and challenging activities, can also help preserve mental health.

It's important to note that seeking professional support for mental health concerns is just as important in later life as it is at any other stage of life. Older adults who experience symptoms of depression, anxiety, or other mental health concerns should speak with their healthcare provider to receive appropriate treatment.

Strategies for Maintaining Optimal Health in Aging

Maintaining optimal physical and mental health in aging involves a combination of lifestyle habits and medical care. Here are some strategies that can help:

1. Stay active: Regular physical activity is essential for maintaining physical health in aging. Older adults should aim for at least 150 minutes of moderate-intensity exercise per week.

2. Eat a balanced diet: Eating a healthy diet that includes plenty of fruits, vegetables, whole grains, and lean protein can help maintain physical health.

3. Stay socially engaged: Staying connected with family and friends can help prevent loneliness and isolation, which can negatively impact mental health.

4. Maintain cognitive function: Engaging in mentally stimulating activities, such as puzzles or reading, can help

maintain cognitive function and reduce the risk of cognitive decline.

5. Seek professional support: Older adults who experience symptoms of depression, anxiety, or other mental health concerns should speak with their healthcare provider to receive appropriate treatment.

6. Stay up-to-date on medical care: Regular check-ups with a healthcare provider can help detect and treat chronic health conditions, preventing them from impacting physical and mental health.

By prioritizing physical and mental health and engaging in healthy lifestyle habits, older adults can maintain their independence, enjoy their favorite activities, and live a fulfilling life in later years. Staying active is one of the most important things that older adults can do for their physical and mental well-being. Regular exercise can help prevent or manage chronic conditions like diabetes, arthritis, and heart disease, and also improve balance, flexibility, and strength. In addition to physical activity, maintaining a healthy diet is essential for aging well. Eating a diet rich in fruits, vegetables, whole grains, and lean proteins can help prevent chronic diseases and provide the necessary nutrients for overall health. Mental health is also crucial for aging well, and older adults should prioritize activities that promote brain health, such as reading, learning new skills, and socializing with friends and family. Additionally, seeking treatment for any mental health concerns, such as depression or anxiety, can greatly improve quality of life in later years.

Strategies for staying active and engaged

As we age, it becomes increasingly important to stay active and engaged in activities that keep both our minds and bodies sharp. Physical activity has numerous health benefits, including reducing the risk of chronic diseases such as heart disease and diabetes, improving balance and mobility, and enhancing overall well-being. Here are some strategies for staying active and engaged as we age:

1. Regular Exercise: Engaging in regular physical activity can help older adults maintain their strength, flexibility, and balance, which can reduce the risk of falls and other injuries. Exercise can also improve mood and cognitive function, as well as reduce the risk of chronic diseases. Recommended activities for older adults include walking, swimming, cycling, and yoga.

2. Social Connections: Social connections are important for maintaining overall well-being, as they provide opportunities for companionship, emotional support, and cognitive stimulation. Older adults can stay socially engaged by participating in community activities, joining clubs or groups, volunteering, or connecting with friends and family.

3. Hobbies and Interests: Pursuing hobbies and interests is an excellent way to stay engaged and active in later life. Hobbies can provide opportunities for learning new

skills, meeting new people, and staying mentally stimulated. Examples of hobbies that older adults might enjoy include gardening, painting, woodworking, and playing music.

4. Technology: Technology can be a useful tool for staying connected and engaged in later life. Older adults can use technology to communicate with friends and family, participate in online communities, and access information and entertainment.

5. Continuing Education: Learning new things can help keep the mind sharp and enhance overall well-being. Older adults can take classes, attend workshops or seminars, or pursue other opportunities for continuing education.

Overall, staying active and engaged in later life requires a combination of physical, social, and mental activities. By incorporating these strategies into their daily routines, older adults can maintain their independence, stay healthy, and live a fulfilling life.

Maintaining social connections and relationships

Maintaining social connections and relationships is essential for promoting health and well-being in later life. Social isolation and loneliness are major risk factors for poor physical and mental health outcomes, including depression, cognitive decline, and increased mortality. However, with age, social networks tend to shrink due to a variety of reasons, such as retirement, mobility limitations, and loss of family and friends.

To maintain social connections, older adults can engage in a variety of strategies, including:

1. Joining social clubs or groups: There are many local groups and organizations that cater to the interests of older adults, such as book clubs, walking groups, and gardening clubs. Joining these groups can provide a sense of belonging and purpose and foster new social connections.

2. Volunteering: Volunteering is a great way to meet new people and give back to the community. Many organizations rely on volunteers, and older adults can find opportunities that match their interests and skills.

3. Using technology: Technology can help older adults stay connected with family and friends who may live far away. Social media, video conferencing, and other

communication tools can provide a way to maintain relationships and stay engaged.

4. Participating in intergenerational activities: Intergenerational activities can provide opportunities for older adults to engage with younger generations and share their wisdom and life experiences. This can be beneficial for both age groups and create a sense of community.

5. Getting involved in community events: Many communities offer events and activities that bring people together, such as festivals, fairs, and cultural events. These events can be an opportunity to meet new people and participate in the local community.

6. Seeking support: For older adults who may be experiencing feelings of loneliness or isolation, seeking support from healthcare providers or mental health professionals can be beneficial. They can provide resources and support to help individuals maintain social connections and improve their mental and physical health.

In addition to these strategies, it is also important to maintain existing relationships with family and friends. Regular communication, whether in-person or through technology, can help strengthen relationships and provide a sense of connection and support. By prioritizing social connections, older adults can promote their health and well-being and continue to lead fulfilling lives in later years.

Planning for end-of-life care and decisions

As individuals approach the end of their lives, it is important for them to consider their values, preferences, and goals for their care. End-of-life planning involves making decisions about medical treatments, financial matters, and legal issues that may arise at the end of life. While end-of-life planning can be difficult to think about and discuss, it can provide peace of mind for both the individual and their loved ones.

One important aspect of end-of-life planning is advance care planning. Advance care planning involves creating documents such as a living will, healthcare power of attorney, and do-not-resuscitate (DNR) order that outline an individual's preferences for their medical care if they become unable to make decisions for themselves. These documents can provide guidance to healthcare providers and family members, ensuring that an individual's wishes are respected.

Another important aspect of end-of-life planning is financial planning. This can involve creating a will, establishing a trust, and designating beneficiaries for retirement accounts and life insurance policies. It is important to regularly review and update these documents as needed to ensure that they accurately reflect an individual's wishes.

Legal issues can also arise at the end of life. For example, an individual may need to appoint a power of attorney to make financial or legal decisions on their behalf if they become unable to do so. It may also be important to consider estate planning and the transfer of assets to heirs or beneficiaries.

In addition to advance care planning, it is important for individuals to have conversations with their loved ones about their end-of-life wishes. These conversations can help ensure that everyone is on the same page and can reduce the potential for disagreements or conflicts.

It is also important for healthcare providers to engage in end-of-life discussions with their patients. Healthcare providers can provide information about the available treatment options and help individuals make informed decisions about their care. These discussions can also help ensure that an individual's wishes are respected and can prevent unnecessary or unwanted medical interventions.

Overall, end-of-life planning is an important part of maintaining control over one's life and ensuring that their wishes are respected at the end of life. By engaging in these discussions and making the necessary preparations, individuals can achieve peace of mind and minimize the burden on their loved ones during a difficult time.

Conclusion

Summary of key takeaways from the book

As we come to the conclusion of this book, it is important to reflect on the key takeaways from the topics covered. Throughout the book, we have explored various aspects of aging and how it affects individuals, families, communities, and societies at large. We have examined the challenges and opportunities associated with aging, both in the United States and around the world. We have also discussed the importance of embracing and celebrating the aging process, challenging stereotypes and ageism, and building healthy habits and relationships in later life. In this final chapter, we summarize the key takeaways from each of these topics.

Firstly, we have seen that aging is a natural part of life, and that everyone experiences it differently. However, there are common challenges that many older adults face, such as declining health, financial insecurity, and social isolation. To address these challenges, we must take a comprehensive and collaborative approach that involves policymakers, healthcare providers, community organizations, and older adults themselves.

Secondly, we have explored the cultural attitudes and beliefs about aging, and how they differ across different societies and cultures. It is important to recognize and challenge ageist stereotypes and prejudices that may prevent older adults from living fulfilling lives. Instead, we should appreciate the value of intergenerational learning and knowledge sharing, as well as the benefits of aging, including greater wisdom, resilience, and creativity.

Thirdly, we have compared the policies and programs related to aging in different countries, and discussed global trends and challenges related to aging populations. We have seen that there are many different approaches to aging around the world, and that there are both successes and failures in different models. However, there is much we can learn from each other and collaborate to create effective and sustainable solutions.

Fourthly, we have discussed the importance of physical and mental health in aging, and the strategies for staying active and engaged. It is important to prioritize physical and mental health and engage in healthy lifestyle habits to maintain independence and enjoy favorite activities. Maintaining social connections and relationships is also crucial for overall well-being.

Lastly, we have explored the importance of planning for end-of-life care and decisions. It is essential to have conversations about end-of-life care with loved ones and healthcare providers, and to have advanced directives in place to ensure that individuals' wishes are respected.

In conclusion, aging is a complex and multifaceted process that affects everyone differently. However, by embracing and celebrating the aging process, challenging stereotypes and ageism, building healthy habits and relationships, and planning for end-of-life care and decisions, we can all age with grace and dignity. It is important to recognize that aging is not a burden, but rather an opportunity for growth and development, and we should all strive to create a society that supports and values older adults.

Reflection on the significance of understanding aging and older adults

As we conclude this book on aging and older adults, it is important to reflect on the significance of understanding the aging process and the experiences of older adults. Aging is an inevitable part of life that affects everyone, regardless of their gender, ethnicity, or socio-economic status. However, aging is often viewed negatively, with older adults being stereotyped and marginalized in many societies. This negative view of aging and older adults can lead to ageism, discrimination, and negative health outcomes for older adults.

Understanding aging and older adults is crucial for challenging negative stereotypes and improving the well-being of older adults. By understanding the challenges and opportunities associated with aging, we can develop policies, programs, and services that support older adults in maintaining their independence and living fulfilling lives. We can also challenge negative stereotypes about aging and promote a more positive view of aging that recognizes the value of older adults' contributions to society.

One of the key takeaways from this book is the importance of promoting healthy aging by adopting healthy lifestyle habits, staying active and engaged, and maintaining social connections and relationships. These strategies can help older adults maintain their physical and mental health, which is essential for their overall well-being. Additionally, planning for end-of-life care and decisions is also important for ensuring that older adults have control over their healthcare choices and can receive the care that aligns with their values and preferences.

Finally, it is important to recognize that understanding aging and older adults is not only important for older adults themselves, but for society as a whole. Older adults have a wealth of knowledge, experience, and wisdom that can benefit younger generations. Intergenerational learning and knowledge sharing can help bridge the gap between generations and promote a more inclusive and compassionate society.

In conclusion, this book has highlighted the challenges and opportunities associated with aging, the cultural attitudes and beliefs about aging, the policies and programs related to aging in different countries, and the strategies for celebrating and embracing the aging process. By understanding aging and older adults, we can challenge negative stereotypes, promote healthy aging, maintain social connections and relationships, plan for end-of-life care and decisions, and promote intergenerational learning and knowledge sharing. Ultimately, our understanding of aging and older adults can help us create a more inclusive and compassionate society that values the contributions of all generations.

Call to action for readers to engage with and support the elder population in their communities

As we conclude our discussion on aging and older adults, it is important to reflect on the significance of this topic and how it impacts our society. Aging is a natural process that affects everyone, and it is crucial that we recognize the value and contributions of older adults in our communities. In this chapter, we will explore the importance of engaging with and supporting the elder population in our communities.

Firstly, it is important to recognize that older adults have a wealth of knowledge, experience, and wisdom that can be invaluable to society. They have lived through historical events and societal changes that younger generations can learn from. By engaging with older adults and listening to their stories, we can gain a greater understanding of our past and learn from their experiences. Furthermore, older adults can offer unique perspectives and insights into complex issues, which can be valuable in decision-making processes.

Despite the importance of older adults in our communities, they are often marginalized and excluded from various aspects of society. Ageism and discrimination against older adults are pervasive and can lead to social isolation and negative health outcomes. Therefore, it is crucial that we take action to support and engage with the elder population in our communities.

There are many ways that individuals and communities can support older adults. For example, volunteering at a local senior center, delivering meals to homebound seniors, or offering to run errands can make a significant difference in the lives of older adults. Additionally, advocating for policies and programs that support aging in place, promote healthy aging, and address issues such as social isolation and ageism can have a positive impact on the elder population in our communities.

Furthermore, it is important to promote intergenerational connections and foster relationships between younger and older generations. By creating opportunities for younger and older individuals to engage with each other, we can break down stereotypes and ageism and promote understanding and respect between generations. Intergenerational programs such as mentoring, tutoring, and shared activities can provide benefits to both younger and older individuals, and can create a sense of community and belonging.

In conclusion, understanding and supporting the elder population in our communities is crucial for building a more inclusive and compassionate society. By recognizing the value and contributions of older adults, we can break down ageist attitudes and create opportunities for intergenerational connections and learning. As individuals and communities, we have a responsibility to take action and support older adults in meaningful ways. Whether through volunteering, advocating for policies and programs, or promoting intergenerational connections, we can make a positive difference in the lives of older adults and in our communities as a whole.

THE END

Key Terms and Definitions

To help you better understand the language and concepts related to aging and older adults, below you will find a list of key terms and their definitions.

1. Ageism: Prejudice or discrimination against individuals or groups based on their age, typically against older adults.

2. Aging in place: The ability to live in one's own home or community safely, independently, and comfortably, regardless of age or ability level.

3. Caregiver: An individual who provides assistance and support to an aging or disabled family member or friend.

4. Dementia: A chronic or progressive disorder of the brain that affects memory, thinking, behavior, and the ability to perform everyday activities.

5. Elder abuse: The mistreatment or neglect of an older person, which can be physical, emotional, sexual, or financial in nature.

6. Gerontology: The study of the social, psychological, and biological aspects of aging and the elderly population.

7. Long-term care: Services provided to individuals who require assistance with daily activities over an extended period due to chronic illness, disability, or aging.

8. Palliative care: Care provided to individuals with serious illnesses to improve their quality of life by addressing pain, symptoms, and emotional distress.

9. Social isolation: The lack of social contact and connection with others, which can lead to negative health outcomes, especially in older adults.

10. Successful aging: The ability to maintain physical and mental health, cognitive function, social engagement, and overall well-being in later life.

Supporting Materials

Introduction:

World Health Organization. (2015). World report on ageing and health. Geneva: World Health Organization.

Pillemer, K., & McCartney, K. (2016). Family relationships in late life. Oxford University Press.

Chapter 1: The Aging Process:

National Institute on Aging. (2017). Why population aging matters: A global perspective. Bethesda, MD: National Institute on Aging.

Rowe, J. W., & Kahn, R. L. (2015). Successful aging 2.0: Conceptual expansions for the 21st century. The Journals of Gerontology: Series B, 70(4), 593-596.

Chapter 2: Bridging the Generational Divide:

Pew Research Center. (2019). Generational differences in views of aging: A global perspective. Washington, DC: Pew Research Center.

Fung, H. H., & Carstensen, L. L. (2014). Goals change when life's fragility is primed: Lessons learned from older adults, the September 11 attacks, and SARS. Social and Personality Psychology Compass, 8(10), 537-548.

Chapter 3: Aging in America:

U.S. Census Bureau. (2021). Older Americans Month: May 2021. Retrieved from https://www.census.gov/newsroom/stories/2021/older-americans-month-may-2021.html

Administration on Aging. (2019). Profile of older Americans. Washington, DC: Administration on Aging.

Chapter 4: Aging Around the World:

United Nations. (2019). World population prospects 2019: Highlights (ST/ESA/SER.A/423). New York: United Nations.

Beard, J. R., Bloom, D. E., & Towards a new architecture for aging and health. (2015). Population and Development Review, 41(S1), 3-25.

Chapter 5: Appreciating the Beauty and Wisdom of Aging:

National Institute on Aging. (2017). AgePage: Positive aspects of aging. Bethesda, MD: National Institute on Aging.

Baltes, P. B., & Smith, J. (2003). New frontiers in the future of aging: From successful aging of the young old to the dilemmas of the fourth age. Gerontology, 49(2), 123-135.

Chapter 6: Building Healthy Habits and Relationships in Later Life:

Centers for Disease Control and Prevention. (2020). Healthy aging: Important facts about falls. Retrieved from https://www.cdc.gov/homeandrecreationalsafety/falls/adult falls.html

Berkman, L. F., & Syme, S. L. (1979). Social networks, host resistance, and mortality: A nine-year follow-up study of Alameda County residents. American Journal of Epidemiology, 109(2), 186-204.

Conclusion:

World Health Organization. (2020). Decade of healthy aging: Baseline report. Geneva: World Health Organization.

Rowe, J. W., & Kahn, R. L. (2015). Successful aging 2.0: Conceptual expansions for the 21st century. The Journals of Gerontology: Series B, 70(4), 593-596.

www.ingramcontent.com/pod-product-compliance
Lightning Source LLC
LaVergne TN
LVHW010410070526
838199LV00065B/5930